# TEETH WHITENING:

# Maintaining a Bright & Radiant Smile

By

Maxwell Angelou

# Table Of Contents

- **Fruits and vegetables**

## Chapter 4: Over-the-Counter Teeth Whitening Products

- **Whitening toothpaste**

- **Whitening strips**

- **Whitening gels**

- **Whitening pens**

## Chapter 5: Professional Teeth Whitening Treatments

- **In-office whitening**

- **At-home whitening kits prescribed by a dentist**

- **Custom-fitted whitening trays**

## Chapter 6: Maintaining Whitened Teeth

- **Oral hygiene tips**

- **Dietary recommendations**

- **Avoiding teeth-staining substances**

- **Follow-up whitening treatments**

## Chapter 7: FAQs About Teeth Whitening

- How often should I whiten my teeth?

- Will teeth whitening cause sensitivity?

- Can I whiten my teeth if I have dental restorations?

- Is teeth whitening safe during pregnancy or breastfeeding?

- How much does teeth whitening cost?

## Chapter 8: Conclusion

- Summary of teeth whitening methods and tips

- Final thoughts and recommendations.

# Chapter 1: Introduction

## Importance of a bright smile

A bright smile is more than just a cosmetic feature; it can also have a significant impact on one's overall health and well-being. A bright smile can boost confidence, improve self-esteem, and enhance personal relationships. This article will explore the importance of a bright smile in detail and how it can positively impact an individual's life.

Firstly, a bright smile can help boost confidence and self-esteem. When someone has a brighter smile, they are more likely to feel confident in their appearance and are more comfortable interacting with others. This increased confidence can have a positive impact on their personal and professional life. For example, in a job interview, a confident and self-assured candidate is more likely to impress the interviewer and land the job.

Secondly, a bright smile can also lead to better oral health. Maintaining a bright smile requires proper dental hygiene, such as brushing twice a day, flossing, and regular visits to the dentist. These habits not only keep teeth white but also help prevent tooth decay and gum disease. Additionally, regular dental check-ups can help detect oral health issues early, preventing them from becoming more serious and costly to treat.

Thirdly, a bright smile can improve personal relationships. Smiling is an important part of human communication, and a bright smile can make a significant difference in how people interact with each other. Smiling can create a positive and welcoming atmosphere, making it easier to form connections with others. A bright smile can also make people more approachable, which is particularly important in social situations.

Fourthly, a bright smile can have a positive impact on mental health. When someone feels confident and happy with their appearance, it can improve their mood and reduce feelings of anxiety or depression. This can lead to improved mental health and overall well-being.

Fifthly, a bright smile can lead to increased success in professional life. In many industries, having a good appearance is essential to success. A bright smile can help create a positive first impression, which can be crucial in business settings. Additionally, a bright smile can convey professionalism and attention to detail, which are important traits in many professions.

Lastly, a bright smile can be an indicator of good overall health. Teeth discoloration can be a sign of underlying health issues, such as poor nutrition, smoking, or other habits that affect overall health. A bright smile, on the other hand, can indicate good overall health and well-being.

In conclusion, a bright smile is more than just a cosmetic feature; it can positively impact an individual's confidence, oral health, personal relationships, mental health, professional success, and overall health. Maintaining a bright smile requires proper dental hygiene and regular visits to the dentist. With a bright smile, individuals can enjoy a happier, healthier, and more fulfilling life.

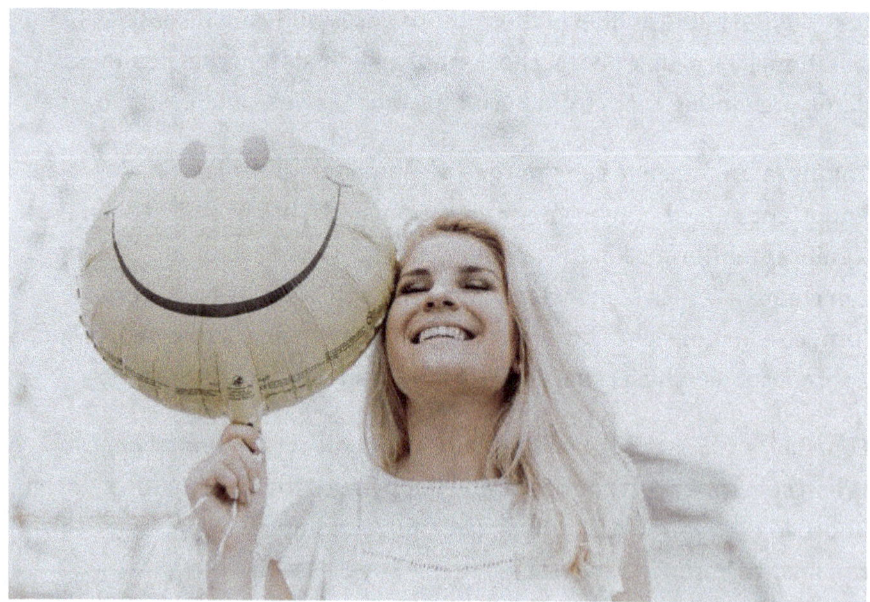

# Factors that cause teeth discoloration

Teeth discoloration can occur due to various factors, including extrinsic factors and intrinsic factors. Extrinsic factors refer to external factors that affect the tooth's enamel, while intrinsic factors refer to internal factors that affect the tooth's dentin.

Here are some of the most common factors that cause teeth discoloration:

- Food and drink: Certain foods and drinks can cause tooth discoloration, especially those that are high in pigment or acidity. Examples include coffee, tea, red wine, berries, tomato sauce, and dark-colored soda.

- Tobacco use: Smoking or chewing tobacco can cause teeth to yellow or brown due to the nicotine and tar content.

- Poor oral hygiene: Inadequate brushing and flossing can lead to the buildup of plaque and tartar, which can cause teeth to appear yellow or brown.

- Aging: As we age, our enamel thins, and our teeth naturally yellow, making them appear less bright.

- **Medications:** Certain medications, such as tetracycline antibiotics, can cause teeth discoloration if taken during tooth development, such as in childhood.

- **Trauma:** Trauma to the tooth, such as a fall or injury, can cause the tooth to darken or become discolored.

- **Genetics:** Some people are more susceptible to tooth discoloration due to genetics, such as having naturally thin or translucent enamel.

- **Fluorosis:** Fluorosis occurs when too much fluoride is ingested during tooth development, causing white or brown discoloration.

- **Health conditions:** Certain health conditions, such as celiac disease, can cause tooth discoloration due to malabsorption of nutrients.

- **Excessive fluoride:** While fluoride is beneficial in preventing tooth decay, excessive fluoride consumption can cause teeth to appear brownish-yellow.

- **Chemotherapy and radiation:** Chemotherapy and radiation treatments can cause teeth discoloration as a side effect.

- **Grinding or clenching:** Habitual grinding or clenching of teeth, known as bruxism, can cause enamel to wear down, making teeth appear yellow or brown.

- **Environmental factors:** Exposure to certain environmental factors, such as high levels of metals like iron or copper, can cause tooth discoloration.

- **Poor nutrition:** A diet lacking in essential vitamins and minerals can cause teeth to appear discolored.

- **Certain dental procedures:** Some dental procedures, such as root canals, can cause teeth to appear grayish or yellow.

- **Illegal drug use:** Certain illegal drugs, such as methamphetamine, can cause severe tooth discoloration, decay, and erosion.

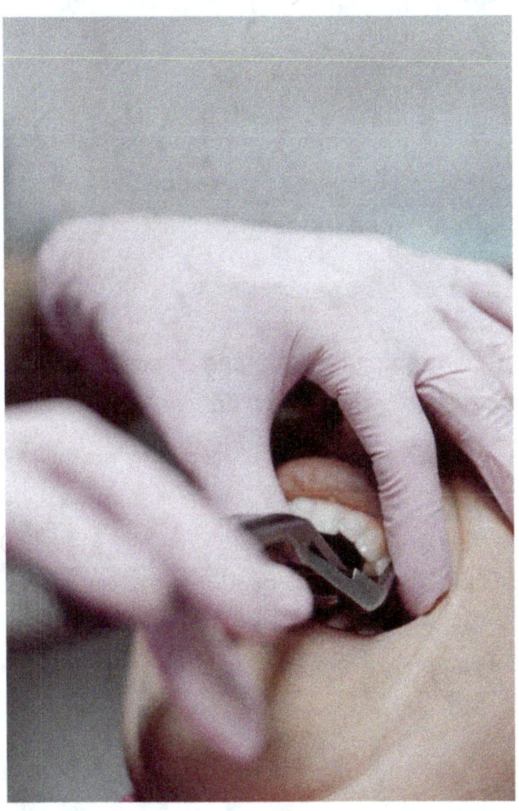

# Benefits of teeth whitening

Teeth whitening is a cosmetic dental procedure that involves removing stains and discoloration from teeth to improve their appearance. Here are some of the benefits of teeth whitening:

- Boosts confidence: A bright, white smile can boost self-esteem and confidence, making individuals feel better about their appearance and improving their overall mental health.

- Improves appearance: Teeth whitening can remove stains and discoloration, making teeth look brighter and more youthful.

- Removes surface stains: Teeth whitening can remove surface stains caused by coffee, tea, tobacco, and other substances that can leave unsightly discoloration on the teeth.

- Safe and effective: Teeth whitening is a safe and effective way to improve the appearance of teeth and can be done in a dentist's office or at home with over-the-counter products.

- Quick and convenient: Teeth whitening procedures are typically quick and convenient, with in-office treatments taking only about an hour, and at-home treatments taking a few days to a few weeks.

- Cost-effective: Teeth whitening is an affordable cosmetic dental procedure that can improve the appearance of teeth without the need for more expensive treatments such as veneers or crowns.

- Reverses the effects of aging: As we age, our teeth naturally yellow and darken. Teeth whitening can help reverse these effects and restore the appearance of a brighter, more youthful smile.

- Promotes good oral hygiene: Teeth whitening can encourage individuals to take better care of their teeth and practice good oral hygiene to maintain the results.

- Makes a great first impression: A bright, white smile can make a great first impression and can be especially beneficial in professional and social situations.

- Non-invasive: Teeth whitening is a non-invasive procedure that does not require any injections or surgery, making it a popular cosmetic dental option.

- Long-lasting results: With proper maintenance and care, teeth whitening results can last for several months to a few years, providing a long-lasting solution for discolored teeth.

- Enhances overall appearance: Teeth whitening can enhance the overall appearance of an individual's face by making teeth appear brighter and more symmetrical, creating a more attractive smile.

- **Can address multiple dental issues:** Teeth whitening can address a range of dental issues, including yellowing, staining, and discoloration caused by food, drink, and aging.

- **May lead to better oral health:** Teeth whitening may lead to better oral health as it can encourage individuals to practice good oral hygiene habits, such as regular brushing and flossing.

- **Can be customized to individual needs:** Teeth whitening procedures can be customized to the individual needs and preferences of the patient, with options ranging from in-office treatments to at-home whitening kits.

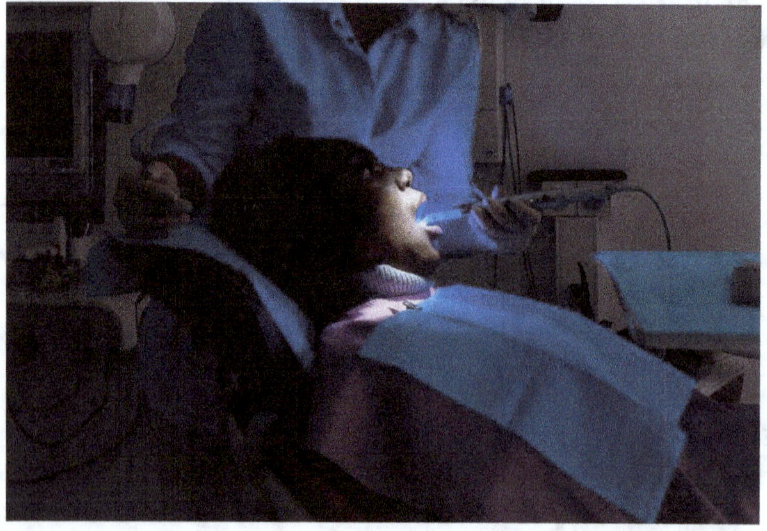

# Chapter 2: Understanding Teeth Whitening

## Types of teeth whitening treatments

There are several types of teeth whitening treatments available, ranging from in-office procedures to at-home kits. Here are some of the most common types of teeth whitening treatments:

- In-office bleaching: In-office bleaching is a professional teeth whitening procedure that is performed in a dental office. The dentist applies a high-concentration bleaching gel to the teeth and uses a special light or laser to activate the gel and accelerate the whitening process. In-office bleaching typically takes one to two hours and can provide immediate and dramatic results.

- At-home bleaching: At-home bleaching involves the use of a custom-made tray and a lower concentration bleaching gel that is worn for a specified period of time each day, typically for a few hours or overnight, for several weeks. At-home bleaching is a more gradual process but can still provide effective results.

- Over-the-counter whitening products: Over-the-counter whitening products include whitening toothpaste, strips, gels, and pens that can be purchased without a prescription. These products typically contain lower concentrations of bleaching agents and may take longer to achieve results than professional whitening treatments.

- **Natural remedies:** Natural remedies for teeth whitening include using baking soda, hydrogen peroxide, and activated charcoal. While these remedies may be effective in removing surface stains, they should be used with caution as they can be abrasive and may cause damage to tooth enamel.

- **Laser teeth whitening:** Laser teeth whitening is a newer technique that uses a laser to activate a whitening gel applied to the teeth. The laser energy accelerates the bleaching process and can provide quick and effective results. However, it can be more expensive than other whitening options.

- **Combination treatments:** Some dental offices offer combination treatments that involve both in-office and at-home whitening. For example, the dentist may perform an in-office bleaching treatment and provide the patient with a custom-made tray and bleaching gel to use at home for maintenance.

- **Zoom whitening:** Zoom whitening is a type of in-office bleaching that uses a special lamp to accelerate the bleaching process. The procedure typically takes about an hour and can provide immediate and dramatic results.

- **Custom-made trays:** Custom-made trays are often used in at-home whitening treatments and are made to fit the patient's teeth precisely. This ensures that the bleaching gel is evenly distributed and that the teeth are whitened evenly.

- **Brush-on whitening:** Brush-on whitening products are similar to whitening pens and can be applied directly to the teeth using a small brush. These products are convenient and easy to use but may not provide as dramatic results as other types of whitening treatments.

- **Internal bleaching:** Internal bleaching is a type of whitening procedure that is used to whiten teeth that have been discolored due to injury or root canal treatment. The bleaching agent is applied directly to the inside of the tooth and left in place for several days to several weeks.

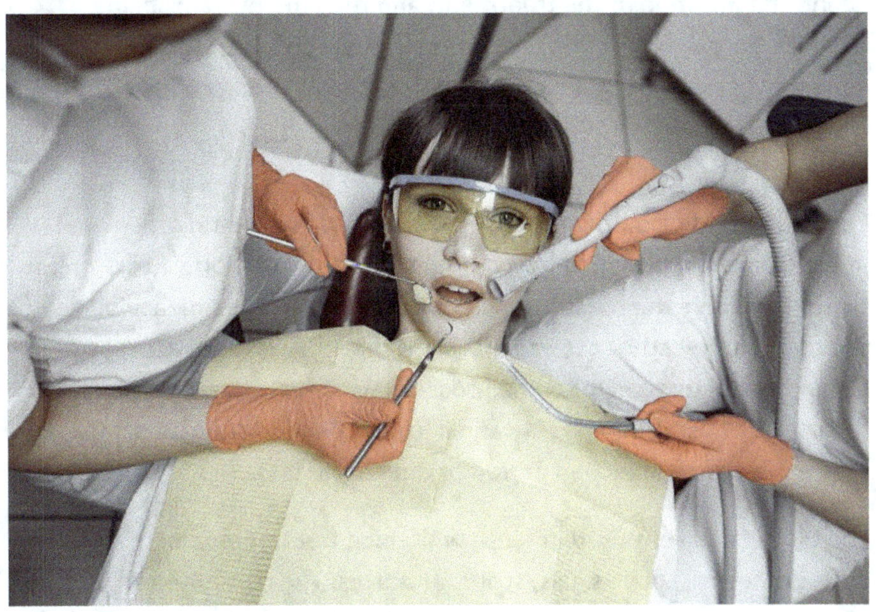

# How teeth whitening works

Teeth whitening works by using a bleaching agent to break down and remove the stains and discoloration that have accumulated on the surface of the teeth. The most common bleaching agents used in teeth whitening treatments are hydrogen peroxide and carbamide peroxide.

When the bleaching agent is applied to the teeth, it penetrates the enamel and begins to break down the complex molecules that have caused the discoloration. The bleaching agent works by breaking down the colored molecules into smaller, less noticeable pieces, making the teeth appear whiter and brighter.

There are several factors that can influence the effectiveness of teeth whitening treatments, including the concentration of the bleaching agent, the duration of the treatment, and the type of stains being treated. For example, surface stains caused by coffee or tobacco are generally easier to remove than stains caused by medications or trauma.

Teeth whitening treatments can be performed in a dental office or at home using a kit provided by a dental professional. In-office treatments typically involve the application of a high-concentration bleaching gel to the teeth, followed by the use of a special light or laser to activate the gel and speed up the whitening process. At-home treatments involve the use of a custom-made tray and a lower concentration bleaching gel that is worn for a specified period of time each day.

The bleaching agent used in teeth whitening treatments can come in different forms, such as gels, strips, or pastes. The concentration of the bleaching agent can also vary depending on the product and the severity of the discoloration being treated.

When the bleaching agent comes into contact with the teeth, it starts to break down the chromogens, which are the pigments that cause discoloration. The bleaching agent enters the tooth enamel and reacts with the chromogens to break them down into smaller, less visible molecules. This process is known as oxidation, and it is what produces the whitening effect.

Different types of stains respond differently to teeth whitening treatments. Surface stains caused by external factors such as food, drinks, and tobacco are generally easier to remove than intrinsic stains that are caused by aging, genetics, or certain medications. Intrinsic stains may require more extensive and prolonged treatments to achieve significant whitening.

Teeth whitening treatments can be performed in a dental office or at home. In-office treatments usually involve the use of high-concentration bleaching agents that are applied to the teeth and activated with a special light or laser. These treatments can produce rapid and dramatic results in a short amount of time, but they can also be more expensive and may cause temporary sensitivity.

At-home teeth whitening kits are also available, which usually involve the use of custom-made trays that are filled with a lower concentration bleaching gel. These trays are worn for a specified amount of time each day, usually for a few weeks, until the desired level of whitening is achieved. At-home treatments are usually less expensive than in-office treatments but can take longer to produce results.

It is important to note that teeth whitening treatments are not permanent and will need to be repeated periodically to maintain the desired level of whiteness. Additionally, teeth whitening treatments may not be suitable for everyone, especially those with existing dental problems such as cavities or gum disease. It is always recommended to consult with a dental professional before starting any teeth whitening treatment.

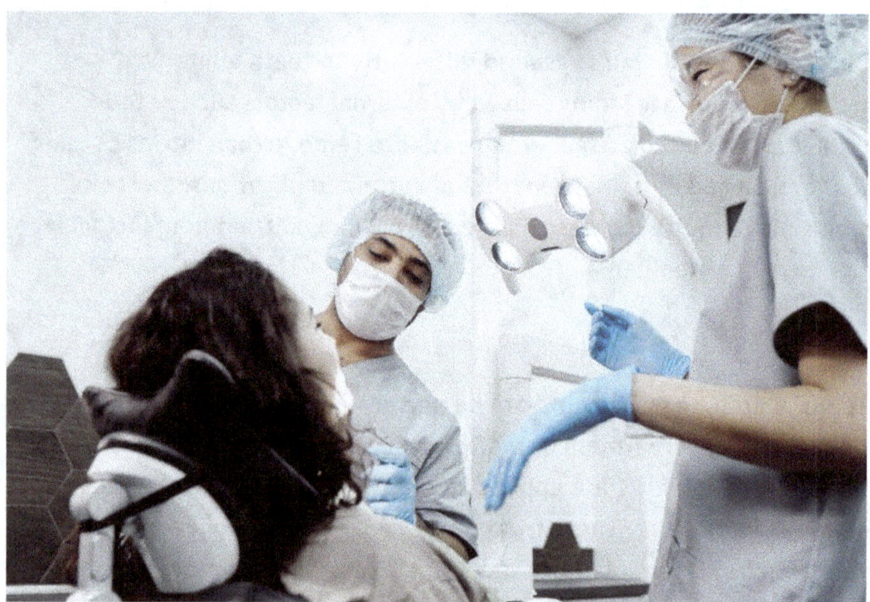

# Risks and side effects of teeth whitening

While teeth whitening is generally considered safe, there are some risks and side effects associated with the procedure. Here are some of the most common ones:

- **Tooth sensitivity: The most common side effect of teeth whitening is tooth sensitivity, which can occur during and after the treatment. This is usually caused by the bleaching agents penetrating the enamel and irritating the nerve endings in the teeth. The sensitivity may be temporary or permanent, depending on the individual and the treatment used.**

- **Gum irritation: The bleaching agents used in teeth whitening treatments can also irritate the gums and cause inflammation, redness, and even bleeding in some cases. This is usually caused by the bleaching agents coming into contact with the soft tissues of the mouth.**

- **Uneven results: Teeth whitening treatments may produce uneven results, especially if they are not applied evenly or if the teeth are naturally uneven in color. This can be particularly noticeable if only some of the teeth are treated.**

- **Relapse: Teeth whitening treatments are not permanent and the effects can diminish over time, especially if the individual continues to consume staining substances such as coffee, tea, or tobacco.**

- **Damage to dental restorations:** Teeth whitening treatments may not be effective on dental restorations such as crowns, veneers, or fillings, and may even damage them if the bleaching agents penetrate the material.

- **Allergic reactions:** Some individuals may have an allergic reaction to the bleaching agents used in teeth whitening treatments, which can cause itching, swelling, or even anaphylaxis in severe cases.

- **Enamel damage:** Overuse of teeth whitening treatments can damage the enamel of the teeth, making them more vulnerable to decay and other dental problems.

- **Root damage:** In rare cases, teeth whitening treatments may cause damage to the roots of the teeth. This can occur if the bleaching agents penetrate too deeply into the tooth, causing irritation and inflammation in the root canal.

- **Discoloration:** In some cases, teeth whitening treatments may actually cause discoloration or blotchiness in the teeth, especially if they are overused or applied incorrectly. This can be difficult to correct and may require additional dental treatments to address.

- **Jaw pain:** Some individuals may experience jaw pain or discomfort during or after teeth whitening treatments. This is usually caused by holding the mouth open for extended periods of time during the treatment.

- **Nausea:** Some individuals may experience nausea or vomiting after teeth whitening treatments, especially if they swallow any of the bleaching agents.

- **Damage to soft tissues:** In rare cases, teeth whitening treatments may cause damage to the soft tissues of the mouth, such as the lips, tongue, or cheeks. This can occur if the bleaching agents come into contact with these tissues and cause irritation or burns.

- **Psychological effects:** While not a physical risk, some individuals may experience psychological effects from teeth whitening treatments, such as an increased focus on their appearance or a heightened sense of self-consciousness about their teeth.

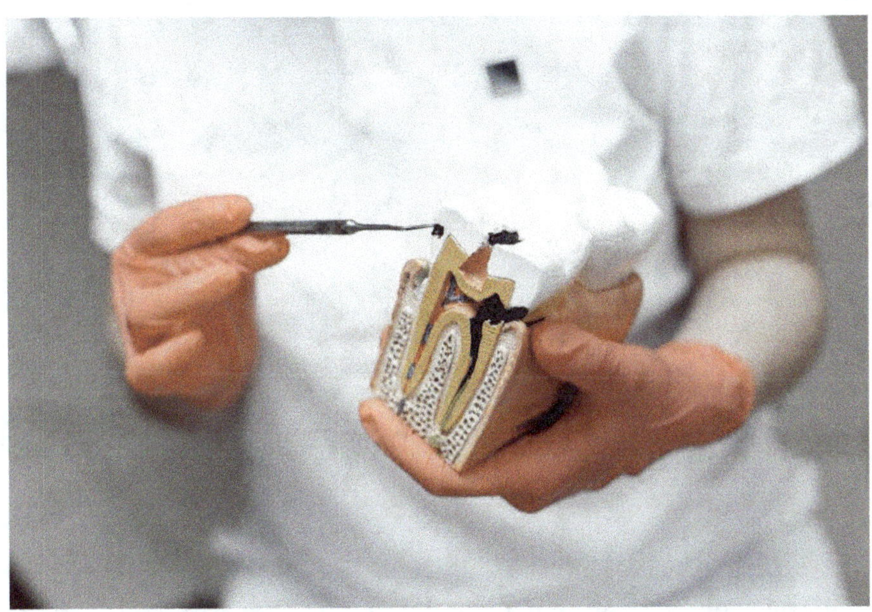

# Chapter 3: Natural Teeth Whitening Methods

## Baking soda

Baking soda is a common household ingredient that has been used for centuries as a natural teeth whitener. Here is a simple method for using baking soda to whiten your teeth naturally:

Ingredients:

- Baking soda

- Water

- Toothbrush

Instructions:

Mix a small amount of baking soda with water to form a paste. Start with a small amount of baking soda (1/4 teaspoon) and add enough water to form a thick paste.

Wet your toothbrush and dip it into the baking soda paste.

Brush your teeth with the baking soda paste for 1-2 minutes, using gentle circular motions.

Spit out the baking soda paste and rinse your mouth with water.

Brush your teeth again with your regular toothpaste to remove any remaining baking soda residue.

Repeat this process once a week to help whiten your teeth naturally.

It is important to note that baking soda can be abrasive and may damage tooth enamel if used excessively or with too much pressure. Therefore, it is recommended to only use this method once a week and to use a gentle touch when brushing with the baking soda paste.

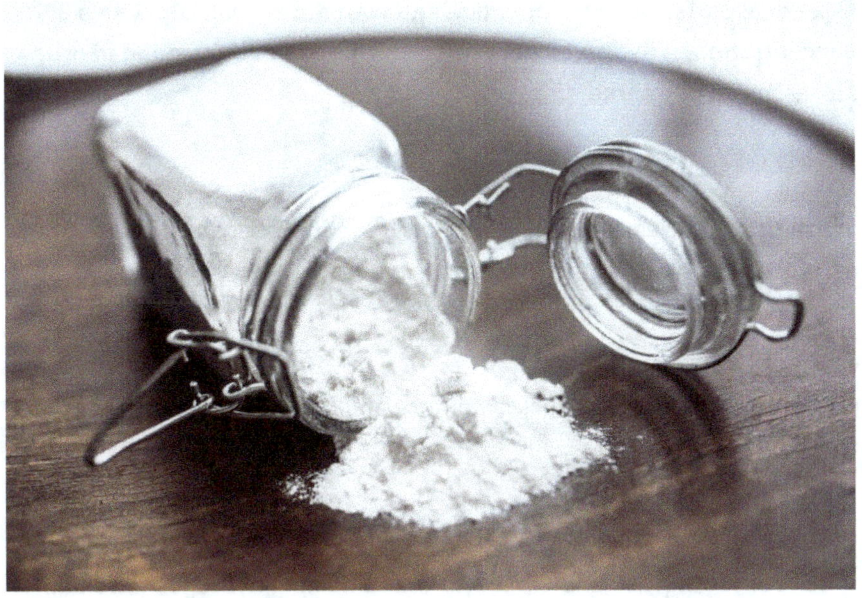

# Hydrogen peroxide

Hydrogen peroxide is another common household ingredient that can be used as a natural teeth whitener. Here is a simple method for using hydrogen peroxide to whiten your teeth naturally:


Ingredients:


Hydrogen peroxide (3% concentration)

Water

Toothbrush

Instructions:


Mix equal parts hydrogen peroxide and water in a small cup. Use a 3% concentration of hydrogen peroxide, which is commonly found in drug stores and supermarkets.


Swish the mixture around in your mouth for 30-60 seconds, being careful not to swallow any of the solution.


Spit out the hydrogen peroxide mixture and rinse your mouth thoroughly with water.

Wet your toothbrush and dip it into the remaining hydrogen peroxide mixture.

Brush your teeth with the hydrogen peroxide mixture for 1-2 minutes, using gentle circular motions.

Spit out the hydrogen peroxide mixture and rinse your mouth with water.

Brush your teeth again with your regular toothpaste to remove any remaining hydrogen peroxide residue.

Repeat this process once a week to help whiten your teeth naturally.

It is important to note that hydrogen peroxide can cause irritation or sensitivity in some individuals, especially if used in high concentrations or for prolonged periods of time. Therefore, it is recommended to use a low concentration of hydrogen peroxide and to follow the instructions carefully.

Additionally, hydrogen peroxide is not recommended for individuals with sensitive teeth or gums, and should be avoided if you have any cuts or sores in your mouth. If you experience any pain or sensitivity while using hydrogen peroxide, stop immediately and rinse your mouth with water.

Overall, hydrogen peroxide can be an effective and affordable way to whiten your teeth naturally, but it is important to use it safely and in moderation to avoid causing damage to your teeth and gums. If you have any concerns or questions about using hydrogen peroxide for teeth whitening, be sure to consult with your dentist or dental hygienist for guidance.

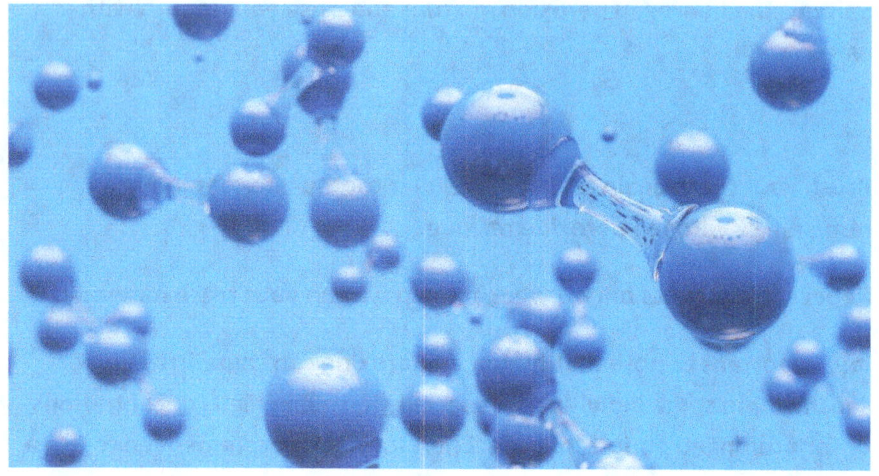

# Coconut oil pulling

Coconut oil pulling is a natural method that has been used for centuries to promote oral health and whiten teeth. Here's how to use coconut oil for teeth whitening:

Ingredients:

Virgin coconut oil

Toothbrush

Instructions:

Put 1-2 tablespoons of virgin coconut oil in your mouth. The oil will solidify at room temperature, so you may need to warm it up in your hands first.

Swish the coconut oil around in your mouth for 15-20 minutes, being careful not to swallow any of the oil.

Spit out the coconut oil and rinse your mouth thoroughly with water.

Brush your teeth as normal with your regular toothpaste.

Repeat this process once a day to help whiten your teeth naturally.

Coconut oil contains lauric acid, which has been shown to have antimicrobial and anti-inflammatory properties that can help promote oral health and prevent plaque buildup. Additionally, swishing the oil around in your mouth can help remove stains and discoloration from your teeth.

It is important to note that coconut oil pulling is not a substitute for regular brushing and flossing, and should be used in combination with a good oral hygiene routine to maintain healthy teeth and gums.

Overall, coconut oil pulling can be an effective and natural way to promote oral health and whiten your teeth, but it may not work for everyone. If you have any concerns or questions about using coconut oil for teeth whitening, be sure to consult with your dentist or dental hygienist for guidance.

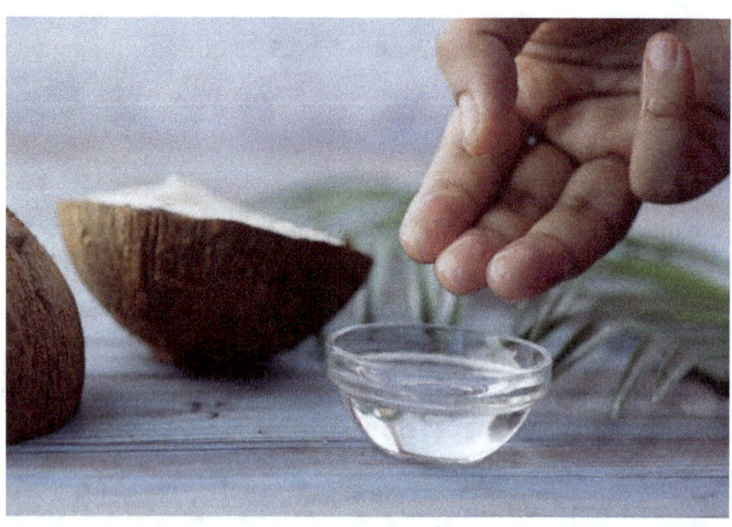

# Activated charcoal

Activated charcoal is a popular natural remedy for teeth whitening due to its ability to absorb and remove surface stains from the teeth. Here's how to use activated charcoal for teeth whitening:

Ingredients:

Activated charcoal powder

Water

Toothbrush

Instructions:

Mix 1-2 teaspoons of activated charcoal powder with a small amount of water to form a thick paste.

Wet your toothbrush and dip it into the activated charcoal paste.

Brush your teeth with the activated charcoal paste for 2-3 minutes, using gentle circular motions.

Spit out the charcoal paste and rinse your mouth thoroughly with water.

Brush your teeth again with your regular toothpaste to remove any remaining charcoal residue.

Repeat this process once or twice a week to help whiten your teeth naturally.

Activated charcoal is highly absorbent and can be messy, so it's important to be careful when using it. It can also be abrasive, so it's recommended to use it only once or twice a week to avoid damaging your enamel.

Additionally, activated charcoal should not be used by individuals with sensitive teeth or gums, and should be avoided if you have any cuts or sores in your mouth. If you experience any pain or sensitivity while using activated charcoal, stop immediately and rinse your mouth with water.

Overall, activated charcoal can be an effective and natural way to remove surface stains from your teeth and promote a brighter smile. However, it is important to use it safely and in moderation to avoid causing damage to your teeth and gums. If you have any concerns or questions about using activated charcoal for teeth whitening, be sure to consult with your dentist or dental hygienist for guidance.

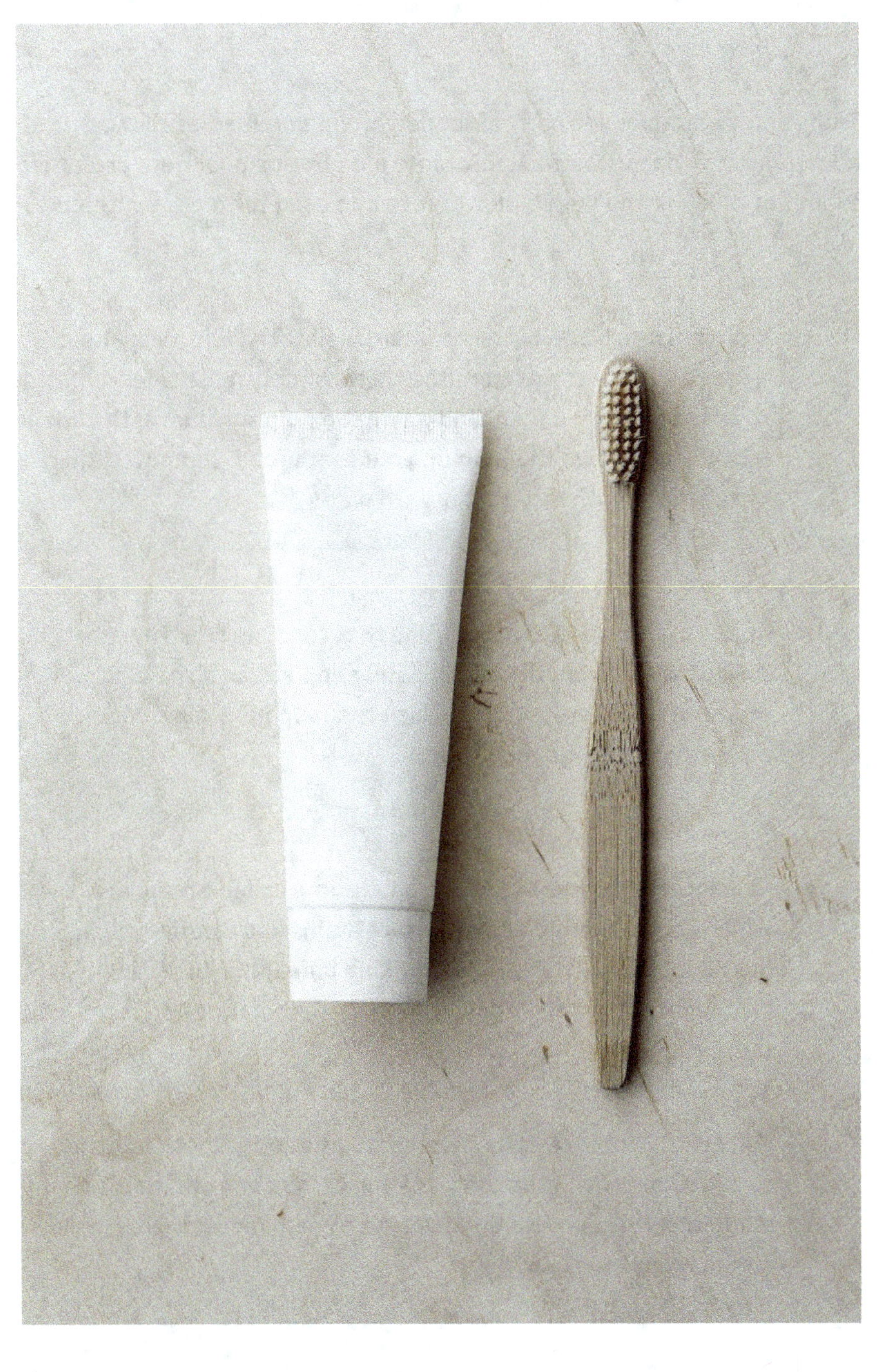

## Fruits and vegetables

Fruits and vegetables are natural teeth whitening remedies that can help remove surface stains and promote a brighter smile. Here are a few examples of fruits and vegetables that can be used for teeth whitening:

- Strawberries: Strawberries contain malic acid, which can help remove surface stains from the teeth. Simply mash a few strawberries into a pulp, and apply the pulp to your teeth with a toothbrush. Leave the pulp on your teeth for 1-2 minutes, then rinse your mouth thoroughly with water.

- Apples: Apples are crunchy fruits that can help scrub away surface stains from the teeth. Eating apples can also help promote saliva production, which can help neutralize bacteria and prevent plaque buildup.

- Pineapple: Pineapple contains an enzyme called bromelain, which can help break down surface stains and remove plaque buildup. Eating pineapple or drinking pineapple juice can help promote oral health and whiten your teeth naturally.

- Carrots: Carrots are crunchy vegetables that can help scrub away surface stains from the teeth. Eating carrots can also help stimulate saliva production, which can help neutralize bacteria and prevent plaque buildup.

- Celery: Celery is another crunchy vegetable that can help scrub away surface stains from the teeth. Eating celery can also help promote saliva production, which can help neutralize bacteria and prevent plaque buildup.

- Baking Soda and Lemon: A mixture of baking soda and lemon can be an effective natural teeth whitening remedy. Baking soda is a mild abrasive that can help remove surface stains from the teeth, while lemon contains citric acid that can help bleach the teeth. To use this remedy, mix a small amount of baking soda with enough freshly squeezed lemon juice to form a paste. Apply the paste to your teeth with a toothbrush and leave it on for 1-2 minutes. Rinse your mouth thoroughly with water and brush your teeth with your regular toothpaste to remove any remaining residue.

- Orange Peel: Orange peel contains a compound called limonene, which can help remove surface stains from the teeth. Simply rub the inside of an orange peel on your teeth for 2-3 minutes, then rinse your mouth thoroughly with water.

- Strawberries and Baking Soda: A mixture of mashed strawberries and baking soda can be an effective natural teeth whitening remedy. Strawberries contain malic acid, which can help remove surface stains from the teeth, while baking soda is a mild abrasive that can help scrub away plaque and tartar. To use this remedy, mash a few strawberries into a pulp, then mix in a small amount of baking soda to form a paste. Apply the paste to your teeth with a toothbrush and leave it on for 5-10 minutes. Rinse your mouth thoroughly with water and brush your teeth with your regular toothpaste to remove any remaining residue.

- Watermelon: Watermelon contains a high amount of water, which can help rinse away food particles and bacteria from the teeth. Eating watermelon can also help promote saliva production, which can help neutralize bacteria and prevent plaque buildup.

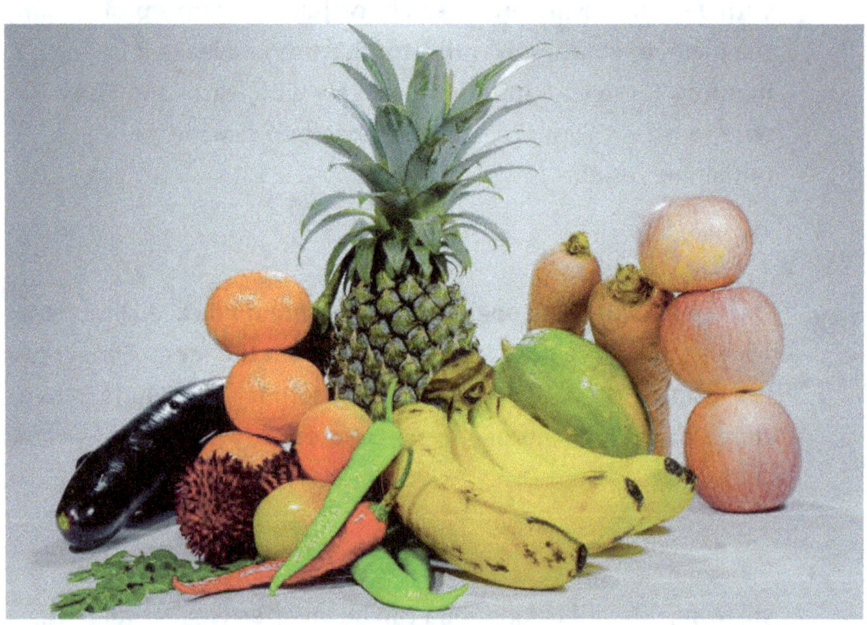

# Chapter 4: Over-the-Counter Teeth Whitening Products

## Whitening toothpaste

Whitening toothpaste is a type of toothpaste that is designed to help remove surface stains from the teeth and provide a brighter, more radiant smile. Unlike traditional toothpaste, whitening toothpaste contains special ingredients that are intended to gently polish and whiten the teeth without causing any damage to the tooth enamel.

The active ingredients in whitening toothpaste may vary, but they typically include abrasive particles like baking soda, silica, or calcium carbonate. These particles work by physically scrubbing away surface stains on the teeth. Additionally, some whitening toothpastes may contain chemical agents like hydrogen peroxide or carbamide peroxide that can help break down and remove deeper stains.

While whitening toothpaste can be an effective way to maintain a brighter smile, it may not provide dramatic results for more severe teeth discoloration. It's important to note that whitening toothpaste does not actually change the natural color of the teeth, but rather removes surface stains to reveal the natural, brighter shade of the teeth.

It's also important to use whitening toothpaste in moderation, as the abrasive particles can potentially damage the tooth enamel if used excessively or aggressively. It's recommended to use whitening toothpaste no more than twice a day, and to talk to your dentist if you have any concerns or questions. Additionally, if you have sensitive teeth, it's important to choose a whitening toothpaste that is specifically designed for sensitive teeth to avoid any discomfort or pain.

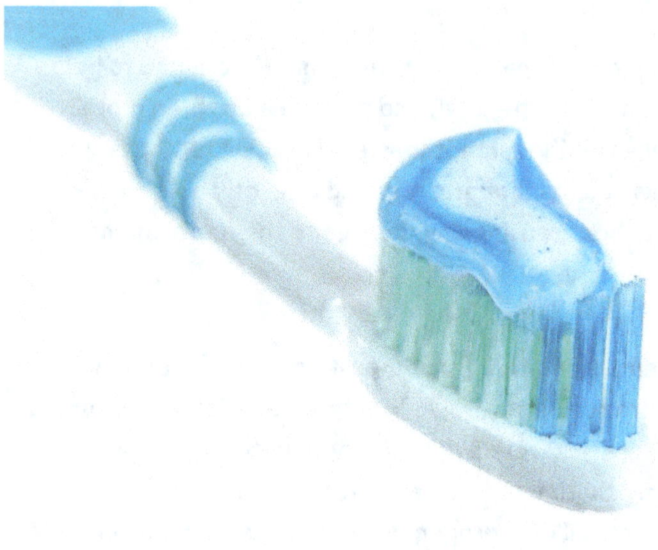

# Whitening strips

Whitening strips are a popular over-the-counter teeth whitening product that can help remove surface stains and provide a brighter smile. These strips typically consist of a thin, flexible plastic strip that is coated with a gel containing hydrogen peroxide or carbamide peroxide, which are the same ingredients used in professional teeth whitening treatments.

To use whitening strips, the user applies the strips to the teeth and allows them to sit for a specified amount of time, usually between 5 and 30 minutes. During this time, the gel penetrates the tooth enamel to break down and remove surface stains.

One of the benefits of whitening strips is that they are relatively easy to use and can be done at home without the need for a dentist visit. They are also typically more affordable than professional teeth whitening treatments.

However, there are some potential risks and side effects associated with using whitening strips. These may include tooth sensitivity or gum irritation, especially if the strips are used too frequently or for too long. Additionally, the strips may not be effective for more severe teeth discoloration, and may not provide the same level of results as professional teeth whitening treatments.

It's important to follow the instructions carefully when using whitening strips and to talk to your dentist if you have any concerns or questions. Your dentist can help determine if whitening strips are a safe and effective option for your individual needs, and can recommend other teeth whitening treatments if necessary.

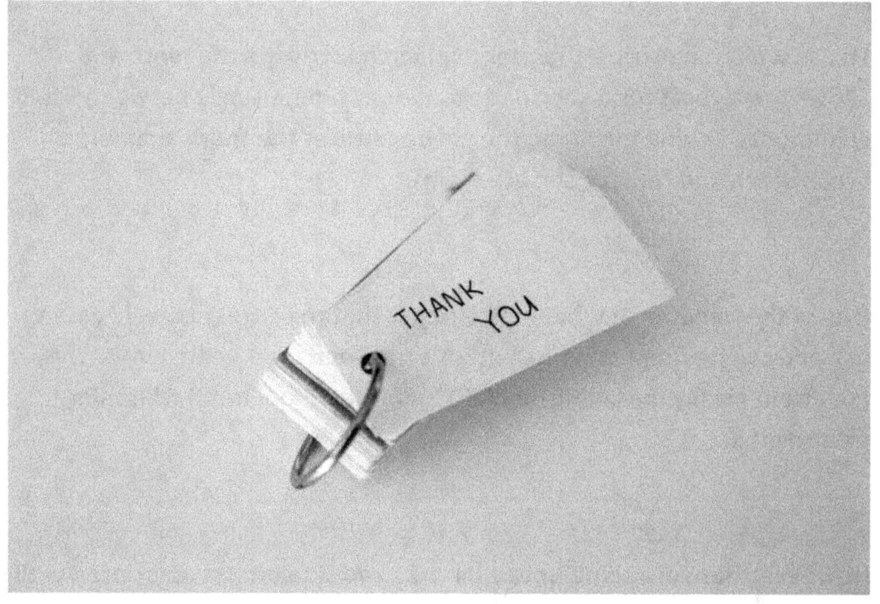

# Whitening gels

Whitening gels are another type of over-the-counter teeth whitening product that can be used to remove surface stains and provide a brighter smile. These gels typically contain hydrogen peroxide or carbamide peroxide, which are the same active ingredients used in professional teeth whitening treatments.

Whitening gels are usually applied to the teeth using a small brush or applicator, and left on for a specified amount of time, usually between 5 and 30 minutes. The gel penetrates the tooth enamel to break down and remove surface stains, revealing a brighter, more radiant smile.

One of the benefits of whitening gels is that they can be more customizable than other types of teeth whitening products, as the user can apply the gel specifically to the areas of the teeth that need the most attention. They can also be more affordable than professional teeth whitening treatments, and can be done at home without the need for a dentist visit.

However, there are some potential risks and side effects associated with using whitening gels. These may include tooth sensitivity or gum irritation, especially if the gel is used too frequently or for too long. Additionally, the gels may not be effective for more severe teeth discoloration, and may not provide the same level of results as professional teeth whitening treatments.

It's important to follow the instructions carefully when using whitening gels and to talk to your dentist if you have any concerns or questions.

Your dentist can help determine if whitening gels are a safe and effective option for your individual needs, and can recommend other teeth whitening treatments if necessary.

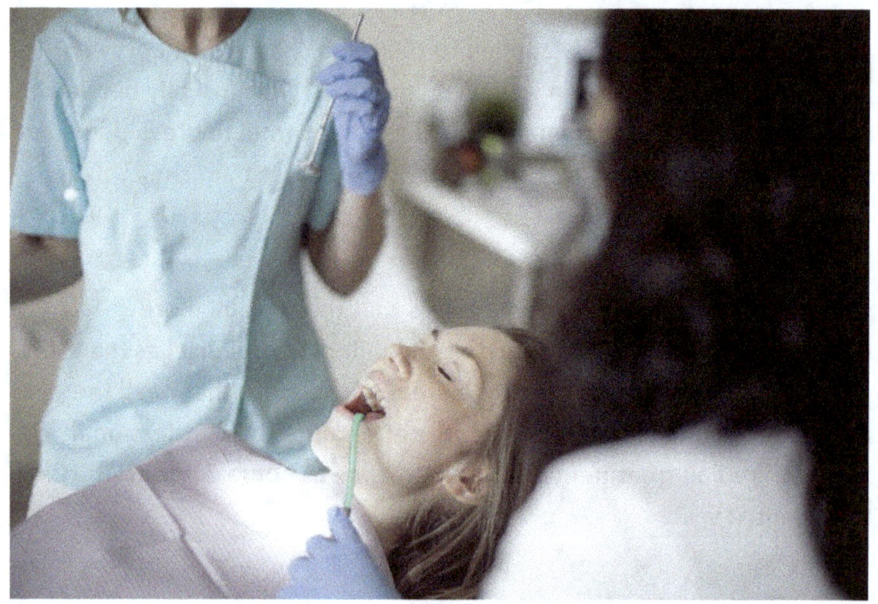

# Whitening pens

Whitening pens are a convenient and easy-to-use type of over-the-counter teeth whitening product that can help remove surface stains and provide a brighter smile. These pens typically consist of a small applicator pen that contains a gel or liquid whitening solution.

To use a whitening pen, the user simply applies the solution to the teeth using the pen applicator, and allows it to dry for a specified amount of time, usually between 30 seconds to a minute. The solution can be left on the teeth or rinsed off after the specified time.

One of the benefits of whitening pens is that they are portable and can be used on-the-go or while traveling. They are also typically more affordable than professional teeth whitening treatments.

However, there are some potential risks and side effects associated with using whitening pens. These may include tooth sensitivity or gum irritation, especially if the solution is used too frequently or for too long. Additionally, the pens may not be effective for more severe teeth discoloration, and may not provide the same level of results as professional teeth whitening treatments.

It's important to follow the instructions carefully when using whitening pens and to talk to your dentist if you have any concerns or questions. Your dentist can help determine if whitening pens are a safe and effective option for your individual needs, and can recommend other teeth whitening treatments if necessary.

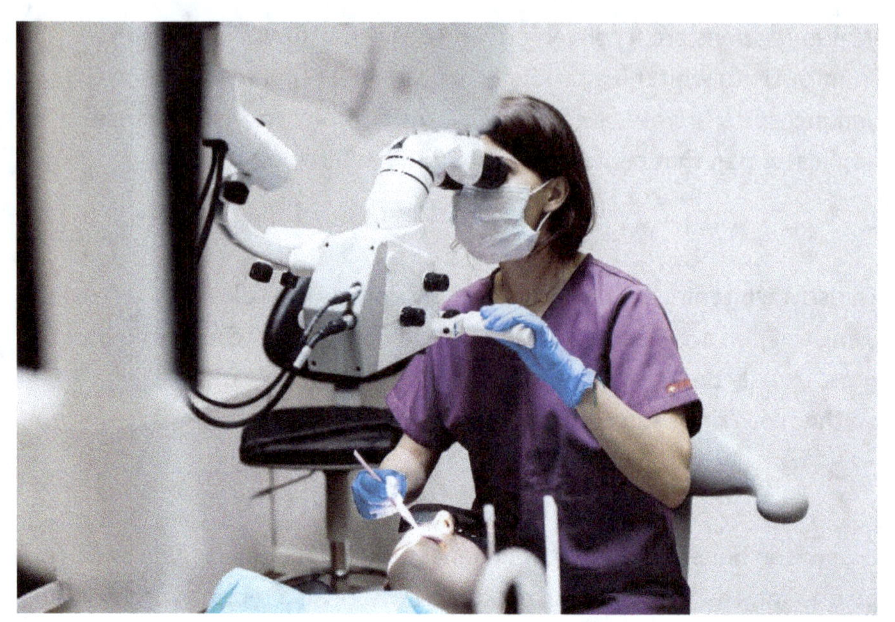

# Chapter 5: Professional Teeth Whitening Treatments

## In-office whitening

In-office teeth whitening is a professional teeth whitening treatment that is performed in a dentist's office. This type of treatment is considered to be the most effective and fastest way to achieve a bright and white smile.

During an in-office teeth whitening treatment, the dentist will first apply a protective gel or shield to the gums to protect them from the whitening solution. Then, a high concentration of hydrogen peroxide or carbamide peroxide gel is applied to the teeth and left on for a specified amount of time, usually between 30 minutes to an hour. The whitening gel is activated using a special light or laser.

The dentist may repeat this process two or three times during the same appointment, depending on the severity of the discoloration and the desired level of whitening.

One of the main benefits of in-office teeth whitening is that it provides immediate and dramatic results. Patients can leave the dentist's office with a significantly whiter and brighter smile in just one visit.

However, there are some potential risks and side effects associated with in-office teeth whitening. These may include tooth sensitivity or gum irritation, especially if the treatment is performed for too long or if the whitening solution is too strong.

In addition, in-office teeth whitening is typically more expensive than over-the-counter teeth whitening products or other professional teeth whitening treatments.

It's important to talk to your dentist about the potential risks and benefits of in-office teeth whitening and to determine if it is the right treatment option for your individual needs. Your dentist may also recommend other teeth whitening treatments, such as at-home whitening trays or whitening strips, depending on your goals and preferences.

Another advantage of in-office teeth whitening is that the treatment is performed under the supervision of a dental professional. This means that the dentist can monitor the patient's progress and adjust the treatment as needed to ensure that the teeth are whitened safely and effectively.

In addition, in-office teeth whitening treatments can be customized to meet the specific needs and preferences of each patient. The dentist can adjust the strength and duration of the whitening solution based on the individual's level of tooth discoloration and sensitivity.

Overall, in-office teeth whitening is a safe and effective way to achieve a brighter and more confident smile. While there are some potential risks and side effects associated with the treatment, these can usually be minimized with proper care and supervision from a dental professional.

# At-home whitening kits prescribed by a dentist

Custom-fitted whitening trays: These are customized trays that are made to fit the patient's teeth perfectly. The dentist will take impressions of the patient's teeth and use them to create a custom tray that will hold the whitening gel in place. The patient will then apply the whitening gel to the tray and wear it for a specified amount of time each day, usually for a few weeks.

Whitening strips: Whitening strips are thin, flexible strips that are coated with a whitening gel. The patient will apply the strips to their teeth and wear them for a specified amount of time each day, usually for a few weeks. Some whitening strips are designed to be worn for only a few minutes at a time, while others may be worn for up to an hour.

Whitening pens: Whitening pens are small, portable pens that contain a whitening gel. The patient will apply the gel directly to their teeth using the pen's applicator tip. Whitening pens are often used for touch-up treatments or to target specific areas of tooth discoloration.

Whitening mouthwash: Whitening mouthwash is a rinse that contains a small amount of hydrogen peroxide or other whitening agents. The patient will rinse their mouth with the mouthwash for a specified amount of time each day, usually for a few weeks.

It's worth noting that at-home whitening kits prescribed by a dentist are typically more effective and safer than over-the-counter options. This is because they are formulated with stronger whitening agents and are often customized to the patient's unique needs.

In addition, dentists may recommend at-home whitening kits for patients who have had in-office whitening treatments in the past but need to touch up their results. At-home kits can help maintain the brightness of the teeth between professional whitening sessions.

It's important to follow the instructions provided by your dentist when using an at-home whitening kit to avoid overuse or misuse of the product. Overuse of whitening products can lead to tooth sensitivity or damage to the enamel, so it's important to use them only as directed.

Overall, at-home whitening kits prescribed by a dentist can be a safe and effective way to achieve a brighter, more confident smile from the comfort of your own home. Consult with your dentist to determine which type of kit is best for you and how to use it properly.

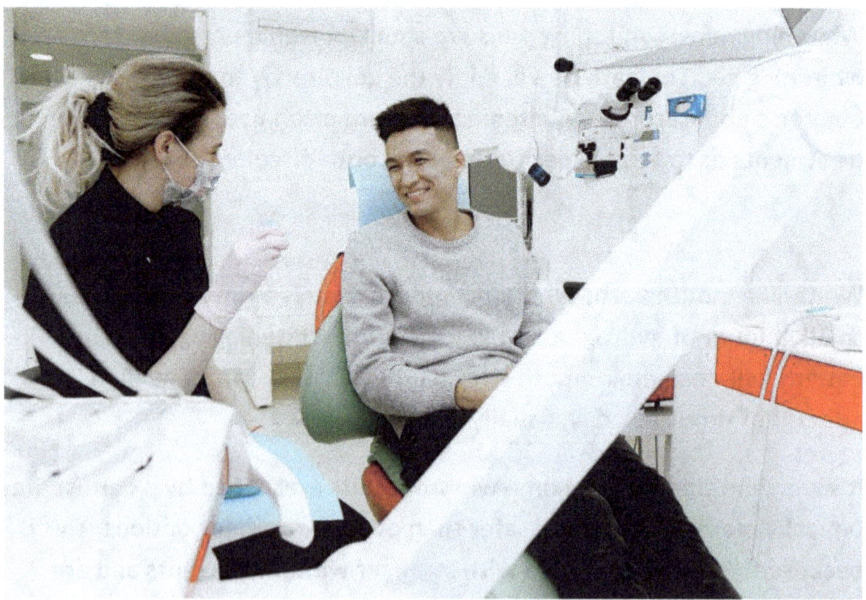

# Custom-fitted whitening trays

- **Opalescence PF:** Opalescence PF is a professional-strength whitening gel that is designed to be used with custom-fitted trays. The gel contains a unique formula that helps to reduce sensitivity and improve the overall health of the teeth while whitening them. Patients can wear the trays for 30 minutes to an hour each day, depending on their desired results.

- **Zoom DayWhite:** Zoom DayWhite is another professional-strength whitening gel that is used with custom-fitted trays. This gel contains a special formula that helps to reduce sensitivity while still providing effective whitening results. Patients can wear the trays for 30 minutes to an hour each day, depending on their desired results.

- **Ultradent Opalescence Go:** Ultradent Opalescence Go is a pre-filled tray system that can be used without the need for custom-fitted trays. The trays are pre-filled with a professional-strength whitening gel and are designed to fit most patients' teeth. The trays can be worn for 15 to 60 minutes each day, depending on the strength of the gel and the patient's desired results.

- **Pola Night:** Pola Night is a professional-strength whitening gel that is used with custom-fitted trays. The gel contains a special formula that helps to reduce sensitivity and improve the overall health of the teeth while whitening them. Patients can wear the trays for 30 minutes to an hour each day, depending on their desired results.

- Custom-fitted whitening trays are designed to fit your teeth precisely, ensuring that the whitening gel is evenly distributed and in contact with all areas of your teeth. This helps to ensure more effective and consistent results compared to over-the-counter whitening options.

- Custom-fitted trays also help to minimize the risk of gum irritation or sensitivity, as the trays are designed to fit snugly around the teeth and avoid contact with the gums. This is important as the whitening gel can cause temporary gum irritation if it comes into contact with the soft tissue.

In addition, custom-fitted trays are often reusable, meaning that you can use them again in the future to touch up your results. This makes them a cost-effective and convenient option for maintaining a brighter, more confident smile.

It's worth noting that custom-fitted trays are typically more expensive than over-the-counter whitening options, as they require a visit to the dentist and the creation of a mold of your teeth. However, many patients find that the results are worth the investment and prefer the convenience and effectiveness of custom-fitted trays over other options.

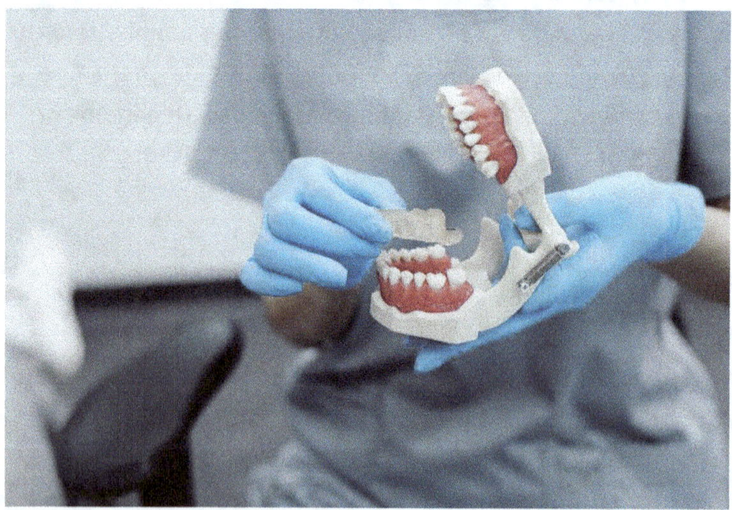

# Chapter 6: Maintaining Whitened Teeth

## Oral hygiene tips

- **Brush twice a day:** Brush your teeth twice a day for two minutes each time using fluoride toothpaste. Use a soft-bristled toothbrush and brush gently in a circular motion to avoid damaging your gums.

- **Floss daily:** Flossing helps to remove plaque and food particles that can't be reached by brushing alone. Use a gentle sawing motion to move the floss between your teeth, and be sure to reach all the way to the gum line.

- **Use mouthwash:** Mouthwash can help to kill bacteria and freshen your breath. Choose an alcohol-free mouthwash that contains fluoride.

- **Drink plenty of water:** Drinking water helps to rinse away food particles and bacteria that can cause tooth decay and bad breath. Aim to drink at least 8 glasses of water each day.

- **Limit sugary and acidic foods and drinks:** Sugary and acidic foods and drinks can erode your enamel and cause tooth decay. Try to limit your intake of these foods and drinks, and brush your teeth or rinse your mouth with water after consuming them.

- **Visit your dentist regularly:** Regular dental check-ups and cleanings are important for maintaining good oral health. Your dentist can identify any issues early on and provide treatment to prevent them from becoming more serious.

- **Quit smoking:** Smoking and using other tobacco products can cause bad breath, stain your teeth, and increase your risk of gum disease and oral cancer. Quitting smoking is one of the best things you can do for your oral and overall health.

- **Eat a healthy diet:** A healthy diet rich in fruits, vegetables, whole grains, and lean proteins can help to provide your body with the nutrients it needs to maintain good oral health. Calcium and vitamin D are particularly important for strong teeth and bones.

- **Use a tongue scraper:** Bacteria can build up on your tongue and cause bad breath. Using a tongue scraper can help to remove this bacteria and freshen your breath.

- **Replace your toothbrush regularly:** Over time, the bristles on your toothbrush can become worn and less effective at removing plaque. Replace your toothbrush every three to four months or sooner if the bristles become frayed.

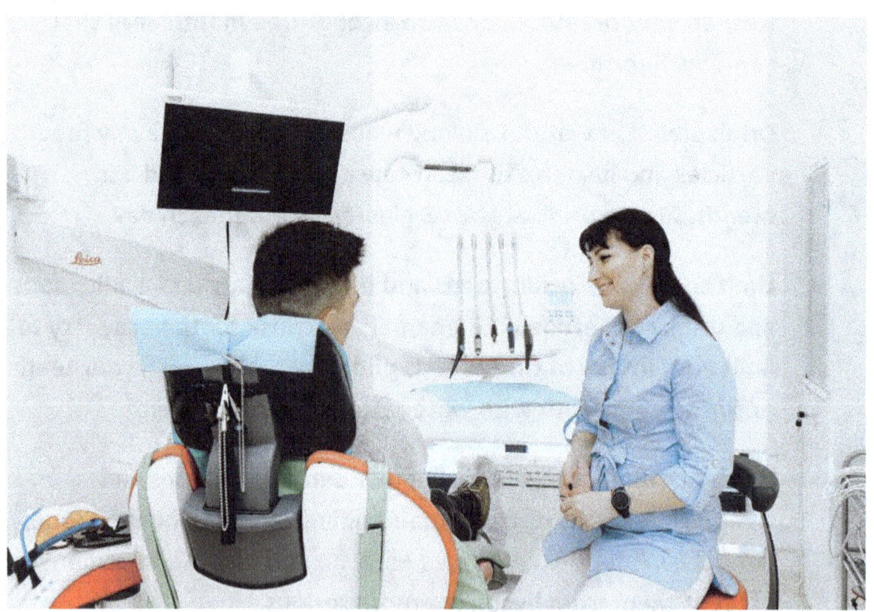

# Dietary recommendations

Diet plays a significant role in maintaining good oral health. Here are some dietary recommendations to help keep your teeth and gums healthy:

- Choose water: Drinking water is important for your overall health, but it's also crucial for your oral health. Water helps to rinse away food particles and bacteria that can cause tooth decay and bad breath. Aim to drink at least 8 glasses of water each day.

- Eat a balanced diet: A balanced diet rich in fruits, vegetables, whole grains, and lean proteins can help to provide your body with the nutrients it needs to maintain good oral health. Calcium and vitamin D are particularly important for strong teeth and bones.

- Avoid sugary and acidic foods and drinks: Sugary and acidic foods and drinks can erode your enamel and cause tooth decay. Try to limit your intake of these foods and drinks, and brush your teeth or rinse your mouth with water after consuming them.

- Choose crunchy fruits and vegetables: Crunchy fruits and vegetables, such as apples, carrots, and celery, can help to clean your teeth and stimulate saliva production, which can neutralize acids in your mouth.

- Avoid snacking between meals: Frequent snacking can increase your risk of tooth decay. When you snack, your mouth produces less saliva, which can allow bacteria to thrive. Try to limit snacking and opt for healthier snack options, such as fruits, vegetables, and nuts.

- **Limit coffee, tea, and wine:** Coffee, tea, and red wine are known to stain teeth. While it's okay to enjoy these beverages in moderation, excessive consumption can lead to discoloration of teeth. If you do indulge, try to rinse your mouth with water after consuming them to minimize their impact on your teeth.

- **Incorporate foods that naturally whiten teeth:** Some foods are known to help naturally whiten teeth. For example, strawberries contain malic acid, which can help to remove surface stains from teeth. Pineapple contains an enzyme called bromelain, which can also help to remove stains. Incorporating these foods into your diet can help to support your oral health and brighten your smile.

- **Chew sugarless gum:** Chewing sugarless gum can help to stimulate saliva production, which can help to neutralize acids in your mouth and prevent tooth decay. Look for gum that contains xylitol, a natural sweetener that can also help to prevent tooth decay.

- **Avoid hard candies and chewy sweets:** Hard candies and chewy sweets can stick to your teeth and increase your risk of tooth decay. If you do indulge, be sure to brush your teeth or rinse your mouth with water afterward.

# Avoiding teeth-staining substances

Certain substances can stain your teeth over time, so it's a good idea to limit your exposure to them as much as possible. Here are some common teeth-staining substances to avoid:

- Tobacco: Smoking or chewing tobacco can cause yellow or brown stains on your teeth. Quitting tobacco use can improve the appearance of your teeth and support better oral health.

- Dark-colored beverages: Coffee, tea, and red wine are all known to stain teeth. If you do indulge, try to drink them through a straw to minimize contact with your teeth. Additionally, rinse your mouth with water after consuming them to reduce their impact.

- Acidic foods and drinks: Acidic foods and drinks, such as citrus fruits, tomato sauce, and vinegar, can erode your tooth enamel and make your teeth more susceptible to staining. If you do consume these foods and drinks, be sure to rinse your mouth with water afterward.

- Dark-colored foods: Certain foods, such as berries and beets, can stain your teeth due to their dark color. While these foods are nutritious, it's a good idea to rinse your mouth with water after consuming them.

- Colored sauces: Sauces such as soy sauce, balsamic vinegar, and curry can stain your teeth over time. If you do consume these sauces, be sure to rinse your mouth with water afterward

- Carbonated drinks: Carbonated drinks such as soda and sports drinks are high in sugar and acid, which can erode your tooth enamel and lead to staining. Try to limit your consumption of these drinks, or switch to sugar-free alternatives.

- Candy and sweets: Hard candy, gummy candy, and other sweets can stick to your teeth and promote bacterial growth, which can lead to staining and decay. If you do indulge, be sure to brush your teeth afterward to remove any residue.

- Poor oral hygiene: Neglecting your oral hygiene routine can lead to a buildup of plaque and bacteria on your teeth, which can cause staining and other dental problems. Be sure to brush your teeth twice a day, floss daily, and visit your dentist regularly for cleanings and checkups.

- Medications: Certain medications, such as tetracycline and doxycycline, can cause staining and discoloration of the teeth. If you're taking any medications, be sure to talk to your dentist about any potential side effects on your teeth.

# Follow-up whitening treatments

After completing a teeth whitening treatment, it's important to take steps to maintain your newly brightened smile. Here are some ways to follow up your whitening treatment:

- **Practice good oral hygiene:** Brush your teeth twice a day with a fluoride toothpaste and floss at least once a day to remove plaque and prevent staining. Consider using a whitening toothpaste to help maintain your new shade.

- **Avoid staining foods and drinks:** To maintain your white smile, it's important to avoid or limit foods and drinks that can stain your teeth, such as coffee, tea, red wine, and dark berries.

- **Use a straw:** When you do indulge in staining beverages, use a straw to minimize contact with your teeth.

- **Rinse your mouth:** After eating or drinking staining substances, rinse your mouth with water to help wash away any residue.

- **Consider touch-up treatments:** Over time, your teeth may start to lose their brightness. If this happens, consider touch-up treatments to maintain your white smile.

- **Visit your dentist regularly:** Regular dental check-ups and cleanings can help prevent staining and maintain your oral health. Your dentist can also advise you on the best ways to maintain your white smile.

- **Use at-home maintenance products:** Your dentist may recommend at-home maintenance products, such as whitening trays or pens, to help maintain your bright smile. Be sure to follow the instructions carefully.

- **Home remedies:** There are a few home remedies that you can try to help maintain your white smile. For example, you can rinse your mouth with a mixture of water and apple cider vinegar or baking soda to help remove surface stains. You can also use a mixture of hydrogen peroxide and baking soda to brush your teeth, but be careful not to overuse this mixture as it can damage your tooth enamel.

- **Wear a nightguard:** If you grind your teeth at night, consider wearing a nightguard to prevent damage to your teeth and maintain your white smile.

- **Be mindful of medications:** Some medications, such as antibiotics and antihistamines, can cause teeth staining. Be mindful of any medications you are taking and talk to your dentist if you have concerns.

# Chapter 7: FAQs About Teeth Whitening

## How often should I whiten my teeth?

The frequency of teeth whitening depends on several factors, including the type of whitening treatment, the severity of the discoloration, and individual preferences. Here are some general guidelines for how often you should whiten your teeth:

- In-office whitening: This type of treatment typically provides the most dramatic results in a single session. Depending on your dentist's recommendation, you may be able to maintain your results with periodic touch-up treatments every six months to a year.

- At-home whitening kits prescribed by a dentist: These kits usually involve wearing custom-fitted trays for a specified period each day for about two weeks. After completing the initial treatment, you may need to use touch-up treatments periodically to maintain your results.

- Over-the-counter whitening products: The frequency of use for these products varies depending on the specific product and the level of whitening desired. Generally, it is recommended to follow the manufacturer's instructions and to avoid overusing the product, which can lead to tooth sensitivity and damage to the enamel.

It is important to note that the frequency of teeth whitening may also depend on your lifestyle habits and dietary choices. For example, if you frequently consume foods and drinks that stain your teeth, such as coffee, tea, and red wine, you may need to whiten your teeth more often. Smoking and tobacco use can also contribute to tooth discoloration and may require more frequent whitening treatments.

However, it is important to balance the desire for a brighter smile with the health of your teeth and gums. Overuse of whitening products or treatments can cause tooth sensitivity, gum irritation, and even damage to the enamel. It is always best to consult with your dentist before starting any whitening regimen to ensure it is safe and appropriate for your dental health.

In addition to regular dental check-ups and professional cleanings, maintaining good oral hygiene habits, such as brushing twice a day and flossing daily, can also help keep your teeth looking bright and healthy. Eating a balanced diet with plenty of fruits and vegetables can also help promote oral health and prevent tooth staining.

# Will teeth whitening cause sensitivity?

Teeth whitening can cause sensitivity in some people, but not everyone experiences it. The sensitivity is usually temporary and can range from mild discomfort to a more intense, sharp pain. The sensitivity occurs because the whitening agents used in teeth whitening treatments can temporarily open up the pores of the teeth, making them more susceptible to external stimuli such as temperature changes.

However, there are steps that can be taken to minimize or prevent sensitivity during and after teeth whitening treatments. These include using a lower concentration of the whitening agent, shorter treatment times, and spacing out treatments over a longer period of time. Your dentist may also recommend using desensitizing toothpaste or other products to help alleviate any sensitivity.

It is important to note that sensitivity is more common with in-office teeth whitening treatments or those that use stronger concentrations of whitening agents. Over-the-counter products such as whitening toothpaste or strips are generally less likely to cause sensitivity. It is always recommended to talk to your dentist before starting any whitening regimen to determine the best course of action for your individual needs and to monitor any potential sensitivity.

# Can I whiten my teeth if I have dental restorations?

If you have dental restorations such as fillings, crowns, bridges, or veneers, it's important to be aware that teeth whitening treatments may not have the same effect on these materials as they do on natural teeth. While natural teeth can be lightened by whitening treatments, dental restorations do not change color with these treatments.

If you have dental restorations and you're considering whitening your teeth, it's important to talk to your dentist first. They can assess the type and location of your dental restorations and help you determine whether teeth whitening is a good option for you. In some cases, they may recommend replacing existing restorations to match your newly whitened teeth.

Additionally, it's important to note that whitening treatments can cause temporary sensitivity in teeth that have dental restorations, as the whitening agents can penetrate the tiny pores in the restorations and affect the underlying tooth structure. In some cases, this sensitivity may be more pronounced than with natural teeth. Your dentist can help you manage any sensitivity and determine the best approach to achieving a brighter smile that's right for you.

# Is teeth whitening safe during pregnancy or breastfeeding?

The safety of teeth whitening during pregnancy or breastfeeding is not yet fully established, and therefore it is generally recommended to avoid teeth whitening treatments during this time. While there is no evidence to suggest that teeth whitening treatments are harmful during pregnancy or breastfeeding, the effects of the treatment on the developing fetus or newborn have not been extensively studied.

Whitening toothpaste and natural remedies, such as oil pulling or activated charcoal, are generally considered safe for use during pregnancy and breastfeeding. However, it is always important to consult with your healthcare provider before using any dental or cosmetic product during pregnancy or while breastfeeding.

If you are pregnant or breastfeeding and you are considering teeth whitening, it is best to wait until after you have given birth or stopped breastfeeding. Your dentist can advise you on the safest and most effective approach to teeth whitening once you have completed this phase of your life.

In addition to the lack of research on the effects of teeth whitening during pregnancy or breastfeeding, there are also concerns about the potential ingestion of the whitening agents. Some whitening products contain hydrogen peroxide or carbamide peroxide, which may be harmful if ingested in large quantities.

During pregnancy, the body undergoes many changes, including hormonal fluctuations that can lead to increased sensitivity in the gums and teeth. This sensitivity may be exacerbated by teeth whitening treatments, potentially causing discomfort or pain.

It is also important to note that dental restorations such as fillings, crowns, and veneers will not whiten along with natural teeth. If you undergo teeth whitening while you have dental restorations, the restorations may appear more noticeable after treatment due to the contrast with the newly whitened natural teeth. In this case, your dentist may recommend replacing the restorations to match the new shade of your teeth.

Overall, while teeth whitening treatments have been shown to be safe and effective for most people, it is important to take precautions during pregnancy and breastfeeding. It is best to discuss your options with your dentist and healthcare provider before undergoing any dental treatment during this time.

# How much does teeth whitening cost?

The cost of teeth whitening can vary depending on the type of treatment you choose and where you live. Here is an overview of the different teeth whitening options and their average costs:

- Whitening Toothpaste: $5-$15 per tube.

- Whitening Strips: $20-$50 per box.

- Whitening Gels: $20-$50 per kit.

- Whitening Pens: $15-$35 per pen.

- Custom-Fitted Whitening Trays: $150-$600.

- In-Office Whitening: $300-$1,000+.

It's important to note that the prices listed above are only averages, and actual costs may vary depending on the location, the dentist, and the level of expertise required.

In-office teeth whitening is typically the most expensive option, but it also tends to produce the most dramatic results. During an in-office treatment, a dentist will apply a high-concentration bleaching gel to your teeth and use a special light to activate the gel. The entire procedure usually takes less than an hour, and you can see results immediately.

Custom-fitted whitening trays are another popular option. With this method, your dentist will take an impression of your teeth and create a set of custom trays for you to wear at home. You will fill the trays with a whitening gel and wear them for a specified amount of time each day, typically for several weeks. While custom trays may take longer to produce noticeable results, they are generally less expensive than in-office treatments.

Whitening strips, gels, and pens are also available for at-home use. These products typically contain lower concentrations of bleaching agents than in-office treatments or custom trays, but they are more affordable and can still produce noticeable results over time.

It's important to note that while over-the-counter whitening products are available at a lower cost, they may not be as effective as professional treatments. Additionally, some people may experience sensitivity or other side effects from using these products. It's always best to consult with your dentist to determine the best whitening option for your specific needs and budget.

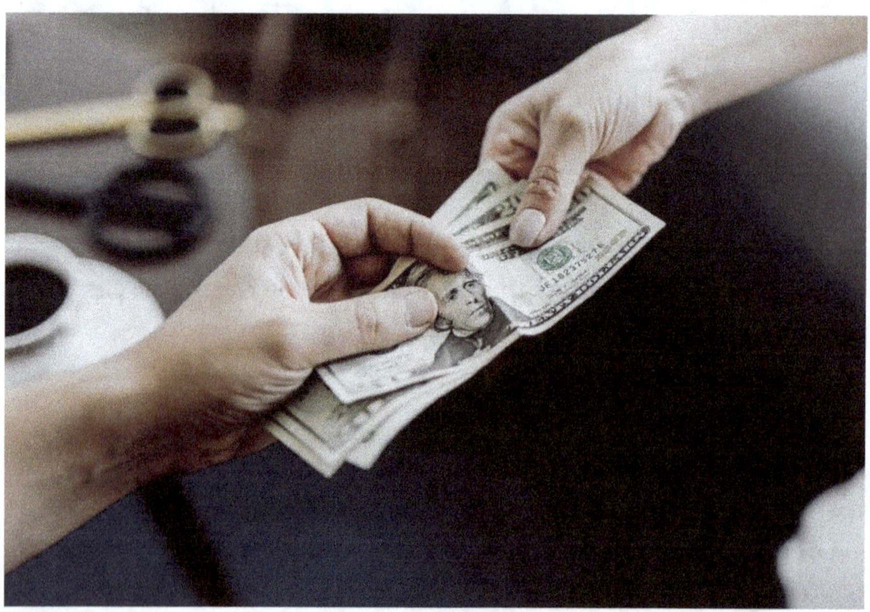

# Chapter 8: Conclusion

## Summary of teeth whitening methods and tips

Teeth whitening is a cosmetic procedure that can enhance the appearance of your teeth by removing discoloration and stains. There are several types of teeth whitening methods available, including at-home kits and in-office treatments. Here are some of the most popular teeth whitening methods:

Whitening toothpaste: This type of toothpaste contains special ingredients that help remove surface stains. It is an easy and affordable way to whiten your teeth, but may not be as effective as other methods.

Whitening strips: These are thin, flexible plastic strips that are coated with a peroxide-based whitening gel. They are applied to the teeth for a specified amount of time each day and can help whiten teeth over several weeks.

Whitening gels: These are peroxide-based gels that are applied directly to the teeth using a brush or tray. They are generally stronger than whitening toothpaste and strips and can provide faster results.

Whitening pens: These are small, pen-like devices that contain a peroxide-based gel. They are applied directly to the teeth and can be used to touch up your smile on the go.

## Summary of teeth whitening methods and tips

In-office whitening: This is the most expensive and effective teeth whitening option. It involves a dentist applying a high-concentration peroxide gel to the teeth, which is activated by a special light. In-office whitening can provide dramatic results in just one visit.

There are also several natural teeth whitening methods, such as using baking soda, hydrogen peroxide, coconut oil pulling, activated charcoal, and fruits and vegetables. These methods are generally safe and affordable, but may not be as effective as professional whitening treatments.

To maintain your newly whitened smile, it is important to practice good oral hygiene habits such as brushing twice a day, flossing daily, and visiting your dentist regularly. It is also recommended to avoid teeth-staining substances like coffee, tea, and tobacco.

Teeth whitening may cause sensitivity in some people, but this can often be managed by using a desensitizing toothpaste or gel. It is also important to talk to your dentist if you have dental restorations or are pregnant or breastfeeding, as teeth whitening may not be recommended in these cases.

The cost of teeth whitening varies depending on the method used and your location. At-home kits can range from $20 to $100, while in-office treatments can cost several hundred dollars or more. It is important to talk to your dentist about the best teeth whitening options for your needs and budget.

# Final thoughts and recommendations

Teeth whitening can be a great way to boost your confidence and improve your overall appearance. There are many different methods and products available, ranging from natural remedies to professional treatments. It is important to consult with your dentist before beginning any whitening treatment to ensure that it is safe for you and to receive personalized recommendations.

In addition to whitening treatments, it is important to maintain good oral hygiene practices and avoid foods and drinks that can stain your teeth. This includes brushing and flossing regularly, using fluoride toothpaste, and scheduling regular dental check-ups and cleanings.

Overall, teeth whitening can be a safe and effective way to improve the appearance of your smile. With proper care and maintenance, you can enjoy a brighter, healthier-looking smile for years to come.

It is also important to keep in mind that teeth whitening may not be effective for everyone. Some people may have intrinsic discoloration or other dental issues that cannot be addressed with whitening treatments alone. In these cases, your dentist may recommend other cosmetic or restorative dental procedures to improve the appearance of your teeth.

When it comes to choosing a teeth whitening method, it is important to consider your personal preferences and lifestyle. Some people may prefer at-home treatments, while others may prefer professional in-office treatments. It is also important to consider the cost of different treatments and whether they fit within your budget.

Ultimately, the most important factor in achieving a bright, healthy-looking smile is to maintain good oral hygiene habits and seek regular dental care. By taking care of your teeth and gums, you can help prevent discoloration and other dental issues and enjoy a beautiful, confident smile for years to come.

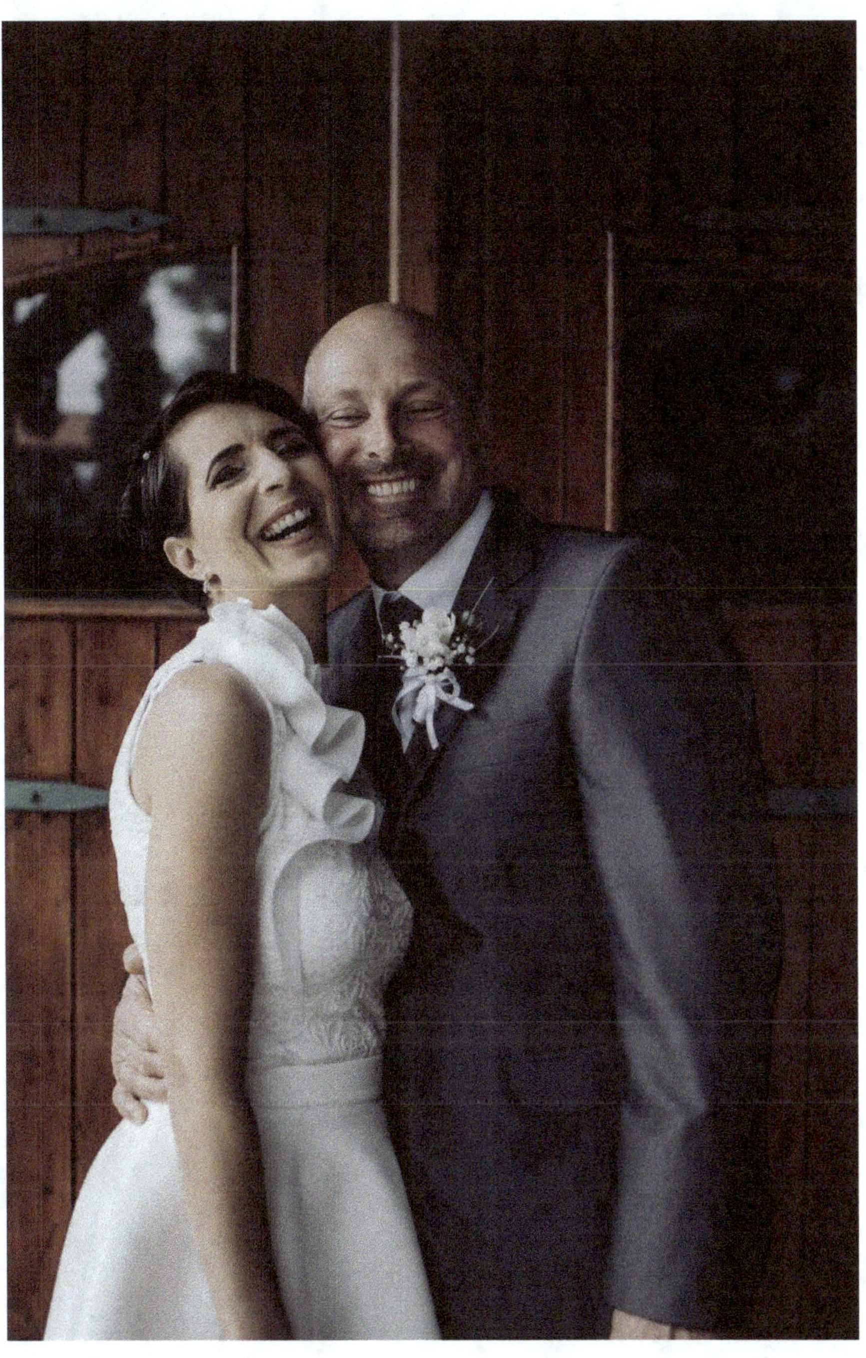

www.ingramcontent.com/pod-product-compliance
Lightning Source LLC
Chambersburg PA
CBHW061604250726
48657CB00017B/1958